First Response Folk Remedies

Quick Old-Fashioned Health Remedies

Compiled and Edited By Debbie Jones

First Edition January 2017

Published by Wild Health Press

© 2017 Debbie Jones

Jones, Debbie, 1939 –

ISBN 978-1542702355

Printed by Create Space, United States of America

TABLE OF CONTENTS

Dyspepsia

Eczema

Eye Problems

Face

Fever

Finger Nails

Flatulance

Freckles

Gout

Hands

Hair

Hangover

Headache

Heart Palpitations

Hiccough

Hoarseness

Indigestion

Insomnia

Jaundice

Leg Cramps

Liver

Loss of Appetite

Mouthwash

Muscular Pains

INTRODUCTION

The information included in this book has been compiled and edited from early newspapers from all over the world.

Before I go any further, I want to make it perfectly clear that these are early folk remedies, whether they actually work or not, there is no scientific evidence for many of them. However, some are more well-known and have been used for many years.

Do not use any of these remedies without checking with your health professional first as medicine has changed and advanced over the past one hundred years and many of these olden-day treatments have been surpassed and may have been dangerous and counter active to the condition trying to be treated. This book is meant as a look back into what early medical treatments were used into various illnesses, and how people coped with these illnesses at the time.

As doctors were so expensive in the early 20th and 19th centuries most people had to come up with their own cures and own ways to cope with illnesses. Many of these treatments are very clever, but we are very lucky these days, in most parts of the world, to have access to effective medications. You could call these early folk remedies 'old wives tales', but sometimes there is something in 'old wives tales'.

In the herb kingdom, one finds remedies almost without number, they are a veritable country apothecary shop in their own right.

I hope you enjoy reading about early folk remedies. Enjoy!

Acne

Spinach has a reputation for clearing the complexion.

Tea tree oil, placed onto pimples when they first appear, helps to dry them out and prevent them from getting larger.

Borax can be used for acne or blackheads. It is taken internally, as well as used in the water for bathing purposes.

Watercress is a destroyer of pimples and a cleanser of the entire system.

Adenoid Problems

Mix three-quarters of a teaspoonful of carbonate of soda and three-quarters of a teaspoonful of salt in a small cup of warm water. If this is used as a gargle and to spray the nostrils it can prevent adenoids in children.

Anaemia

Watercress contains much iron and is a real blood medicine.

Anxiety

Potatoes are good for the nervy person.

Celery tones the nerves. Nervous people should take it in some form, either cooked or raw every day. It can be made very nutty and digestible by peeling away all its stringy fibres if more than the inner heart is eaten. Those who have stormy nerve disorders, such as neuralgia or sciatica, should eat as much celery as possible, in soup as strong celery extract as a vegetable, raw with bread and butter, in all manner of ways so as to get as much variety with it as possible. There is a quality in it that soothes and heals the nerves, and when indigestion is caused by nervous inability to assimilate food, celery will cure it.

Asparagus has a gentle sedative effect for nervousness. This is due to the salts it contains.

Turnips are good for nervous disorders but not in a large quantity as they may cause digestive disturbances.

Asthma

Carrots are excellent for asthma sufferers.

For asthma, mix 1 ounce castor oil with 4 ounces of honey and take one tablespoonful night and morning.

Carrots and turnips act upon the breathing apparatus. Bronchial troubles and asthma are relieved by free use of this diet.

Bed Sores

Olive oil gently rubbed into a spot that begins to look red will prevent bed sores. When bed sores have once formed, brush them gently over with beaten white of egg, and let it dry on. The egg forms a fine skin over the affected part, and gives it a chance to heal.

Biliary Digestion

The specific dietetic value of lemons lies in their potash salts, the citrate, malate, and tartrate, which are antiscorbutic and of assistance in promoting biliary digestion.

Blood

Astringents contract tissue, reduce the size of blood vessels, and coagulates albuminous fluids, checks secretions, mucous discharges, and haemorrhages. Oak bark, raspberry leaves, rosemary, yarrow and wattlebark.

Boils

Apply poultices of bread and milk which will help bring them to a head.

The flowers from the elderberry as an ointment made by mixing them with mutton makes a soothing cream to use on boils.

Bruises

Bathe with hot water night and morning for about half an hour and then bandage after each treatment.

Arnica tincture is a remedy used for bruises. It helps prevent discolouration and reduces swelling.

Wormwood boiled in vinegar and applied as hot as can be taken on a bruise is an invaluable remedy.

Burns

Unless severe, a thick paste of flour and water is good, or white of egg spread over. The object is to exclude the air from the burnt flesh.

Bicarbonate of soda is a splendid dressing for a burn.

Chilblain

Warm brine has a wonderful effect in stopping the irritation of a chilblain.

Colic

When sudden colic was induced by an overloaded stomach, how a cup of warm mustard-water relieved by causing the stomach to throw off its burden.

A cordial made from blackberries is greatly recommended by Devonshire country folk as a cure for colic, and many a farmer's wife makes blackberry cordial.

Constipation

Drinking hot water can help relieve constipation. It should be drunk soon after rising, perhaps half an hour before breakfast. Begin with half a tea-cupful and gradually increase to a tumblerful or even more.

Adding salt to food can assist to prevent constipation.

Two or 3 apples taken at night, either cooked or raw will help with constipation. The malic acid which the apple contains will help eliminate the body of waste.

Carthartics produce movements of the bowels. They are classed as aperient laxatives when their action is mild; purgative when the action is more severe. Laxative – honey, figs, nuts, olive oil, strawberries, tomatoes, raspberries, gooseberries, nuts, salad vegetables, spinach, onions, centuary, dandelion root, rhubarb. Purgative – aloes, senna, castor oil.

Corns

For soft corns a piece of cotton wool saturated with castor oil and placed between the toes, where soft corns are mostly to be found will soon cure them.

Coughs & Colds

The despised prickly pear yields a splendid cough mixture. Rub all the hairs off a leaf and cut up and simmer in water low enough for it to become a thick jelly. When ready, strain and add a little honey and lemon juice. This has been used in cases of whooping cough in the past.

A mustard plaster on the chest will loosen up a cough wonderfully. Also a mustard foot-bath, hot as can be endured taken before going to bed, accompanied by a good hot drink of lemonade (made from lemons), will give good relief.

A gargle of hot water and a small quantity of table salt is very good for breaking up a common cold if taken at the start of the illness.

For a hard cough, a home made syrup from the following recipe is very good – equal parts flaxseed and licorice. After steeping, add equal parts of sugar and molasses, and boil to a thin syrup, Dose, one or two teaspoonfuls.

Another remedy is onion syrup made in this way – a layer of sliced onions, a layer of white sugar, followed by another of onions, then sugar, and so on till the dish is full. Cover and place under a heavy weight. Let it stand several hours till the juice of the onions is well pressed out. Drain off the syrup and give a teaspoonful at a time.

Lemon-sage is also very good in the early stages of colds. This is by using an infusion of sage mixed with hot lemonade (made with lemons).

Another treatment for colds is to use hot water foot baths to which salt and mustard have been added.

Another possible treatment for a cold is a glass of strong and hot whisky taken at the very beginning of the illness and after the sufferer has got into bed.

An old fashioned and very good cure for a cold is a few spoonfuls of black current jam (home made) in a glass of hot water.

Grapes relieve feverish colds by the citric acid they contain.

One of the oldest of country remedies for a cold is mulled elderberry wine, concocted from the fruit with raisins, sugar, and spices. Its efficacy has been attested by generations, and science has provided the explanation that elderberries furnish viburnic acid, a substance which induces sweating and is especially curative of inflammatory bronchial soreness.

For a troublesome cough, put a lemon in a cool oven, leave it until warmed through, then squeeze out the juice, and add sufficient honey to make a thick syrup. Keep it warm and take a teaspoonful when the cough is troublesome.

For feverish cough, a preparation for the cough can be made from the following: honey, olive oil, lemon juice, sweet spirits of nitre, one fluid ounce of each. To be taken several times a day in half fluid drachm doses.

For an obstinate cough: mix equal quantities honey, linseed oil and whisky. Take one tablespoonful three or four times a day.

Elderberry wine heated and mixed with a little cinnamon, is one of the best preventatives known against a chill.

Vinegar, honey and butter mixed in a cup and heated before slipping will cure a sore throat.

Black currant jam made into tea is the old fashioned cure for a cold.

Linseed Tea – When coughs and colds are very prevalent, linseed tea is very easily made. Put six tablespoonfuls of linseed and one quart of water into a pan, and boil it for 10 minutes. Then pour it off, and add to it some slices of lemon and brown sugar to taste. If the flavour of liquorice be liked, an ounce of it may be added. This is a refreshing and very useful drink, especially for children with feverish colds, when there is sure to be much discomfort from thirst.

Corns

Salicylic acid is the infallible cure for corns or rub them with an apple.

A poultice of vinegar and stale bread applied nightly is one of the best dressings for a painful corn.

Cuts

Although sugar has no disinfecting qualities, if it is applied to a clean wound it helps to heal it rapidly.

Diarrhoea

The blackberry is another fruit with valuable medicinal properties. If desiccated in a moderately hot oven and afterwards reduced to powder, it will prove an efficacious remedy for dysentery. A similar effect is produced by an extract of the bilberry, prepared by pouring some good brandy over two handfuls of the fruit in a bottle. Obstinate diarrhoea may be cured by giving doses of a tablespoonful of the extract with a wineglassful of warm water; and repeated at intervals of two hours if needed. It is said that this will prove effectual even in the most severe cases of dysenteric diarrhoea.

Blackberries as a tonic are useful in all forms of diarrhoea.

Bananas, especially if cooked, are useful as a good for those suffering from chronic diarrhoea.

Digestive Disturbances

Buttermilk is excellent for digestive disturbances.

Onion contains a volatile principle, sulphide of allyl, which is acrid and stimulating. It quickens the circulation and assists in digestion.

Demulcents act on the internal lining of the digestive tract, soothing them and protecting them from irritation. Sweet almonds, sago, cornflour, figs, olive oil, egg white, butter, gum acacia, liquorice, marshmallow, slippery elm, colt's foot.

Dry Skin

The best lotion for a dry skin is made of equal parts of rosewater and olive oil, which should be well rubbed in after washing.

Dysentery

The blackberry is another fruit with valuable medicinal properties. If desiccated in a moderately hot oven and afterwards reduced to powder, it will prove an efficacious remedy for dysentery. A similar effect is produced by an extract of the bilberry, prepared by pouring some good brandy over two handfuls of the fruit in a bottle. Obstinate diarrhoea may be cured by giving doses of a tablespoonful of the extract with a wineglassful of warm water; and repeated at intervals of two hours if needed. It is said that this will prove effectual even in the most severe cases of dysenteric diarrhoea.

Dyspepsia

Cider is an excellent remedy for dyspepsia.

Liquorice is an excellent remedy. A little piece of liquorice slowly dissolved in the mouth supplies the stomach with a soothing and protective coat.

Another possible treatment for dyspepsia is a glass of hot water, in which an eggspoonful of salt is dissolved, to be taken fifteen or twenty minutes before meals. Sip it.

Charcoal is another very good cure, it absorbs the gases produced by fermentation of the food.

Eczema

The system is asking for acid. Suck the juice of oranges.

Treat eczema with cornflour.

Oil of the walnut kernel, when applied externally for eczema and other diseased conditions of the skin, can greatly assist.

Eye Problems

Tired eyes - A does of cod liver oil or a cup of warm milk is a help for tired eyes.

Inflamed eyes – A good wash for the eyes when inflamed from cold or loss of sleep is 1 ounce of distilled witch hazel and 1 ounce of pure water. Bathe the eyes frequently with this wash, and the result should be helpful.

Puffy eyes are generally due to some sort of kidney ailment. Cold water should be taken very freely. Make it a practice to drink a glassful half an hour before each meal, and another one or two hours after, and the puffy places will not only vanish, but he complexion will be clearer and the general health much improved.

Face

The best cosmetic in the world is rain water. Bathe the face night and morning with rain water made as hot as can be borne, using a piece of fine flannel instead of a sponge. Rub well, and use neither soap nor powder.

Spinach juice from cooking the leaves without any water is a wholesome drink and improves the complexion. Also the juice of a beetroot is excellent for a complexion improver, but this is a cosmetic, and must be applied with a brush.

If you want a good complexion eat lots of watercress.

Fever

Use hot water foot baths to which salt and mustard have been added.

Oranges allay fever.

Febrifuges or antipyretics reduce and control the temperature in fever. Apple, tea, the juices of elderberry, grapes, oranges, lemons, barley water, limejuice, angelica, boneset, marshmallow, pennyroyal, raspberry leaves, yarrow.

Lemon juice may assist to bring down the temperature of a fever-stricken patient.

Finger Nails

Lemon juice is excellent for keeping the finger nails in good condition. It is a good practice to keep half a lemon in the bathroom or kitchen, and to make a practice of pressing the finger nails into the pulp every time the hands are washed. Lemon juice removes stains from the nails, so that the half-moon is displayed. When lemon juice is employed in this way the finger nails do not split or become brittle.

Flatulance

Carminatives stimulate the muscles of the stomach and intestines, expel gases, and relieve griping. Thyme, angelica seeds, aniseed, fennel, mint and coriander seed.

Grated nutmeg, taken in hot water, will cure a case of flatulence, even occasionally in a case of long standing.

Freckles

By applying the following sulpho-carbolate of lime, 2 ounces; glycerine and rosewater, 35 ounces of each; alcohol 5 ounces. Wash the skin with a little of this lotion twice in twenty-four hours allowing it to remain damp with the lotion for half an hour.

Gout

Spinach is good for gout.

Apples help ward off gout.

Eat a dozen walnuts a day and avoid sweet foods.

Hands

To soften the hands – Take an equal quantity of glycerine and lemon juice. Rub well on the hands, and allow it to dry thoroughly into the skin. This is a good recipe for anyone who is constantly plunging the hands into water or strong disinfectants.

For cracked skin on the hands lemon juice in conjunction with glycerine or milk is a good remedy.

Hair

Brill cream for the hair – Pure glycerine, one ounce; strongest spirits of wine, eight ounces and seven drachms; oil of bergamot one drachin. Shake thoroughly after mixing, and always repeat the shaking before pouring out. A little sprayed over the hair, or applied to the comb before using the latter will increase the lustre and suppleness of the hair.

Hangover

Treatment for a hangover, eat a persimmon before your first drink. This yellowish-red pulpy fruit reduces the amount of acetoaldehyde in the blood stream. This is the substance produced when alcohol is broken down in the body and it is believed that this is the cause of a hangover.

Water is a great cure for a hangover.

Another possible cure for hangover is to take vitamin C and honey which contains levulose.

Passionfruit nectar with dash of bitters.

Black coffee, rum and cream mixed thoroughly.

Pea soup.

Hot potato dumplings.

Freshly sliced pineapple.

Milk helps.

Take aspirin and drink lots of water.

Don't drink!!!

Headache

Essence of Peppermint, applied with the finger tips over the seat of pain, often gives relief in headache and neuralgia. Do not put it directly under the eye as this can cause pain.

Make a very strong cup of tea. Into another cup put six cloves, and pour on about two teaspoonfuls of boiling water. Cover with a saucer. Then make tea. Add cloves and liquid to the cup of tea. Partly chew the cloves as you are sipping your tea. Then lie down for a few minutes. Do not eat immediately after. This works for most headaches – bilious, anxiety, nerves, in around 10 minutes.

For bilious headaches take a glass of very hot water with the juice of half a lemon squeezed into it first thing every morning, and try not to have breakfast for half an hour at the least after it. Common salt taken in liquid form up the nose will give some relief. Rose water mixed with half a pint of rain water, and the eyes bathed in this liquid will help strengthen the nerves and relieve the pain. The pain is caused by, in most cases, not blinking enough which puts strain on the nerves.

Putting the feet in hot water will invariably cure a headache, from whatever cause it arises. The head aches when, from any cause, the little blood vessels in the brain are too full. Putting the feet in hot water draws the blood from the head.

When you feel a headache coming on, add about half a teaspoonful of carbonate of soda to the juice of half a lemon, fill up the glass with water – warm for preference – and drink,

Heart Palpitations

Asparagus has a gentle sedative action on the heart, calming palpitations.

Lemon juice has a sedative effect and allays hysterical palpitations of the heart. For a restless person of ardent temperament and active, plethoric circulation a lemon-squash, unsweetened, of not more than half a tumblerful, is a capital sedative.

Hiccough

For hiccough's press the finger firmly on the upper lip, just under the nose.

Indigestion

A teaspoonful of mustard mixed with a small cupful of water is good for indigestion.

Hoarseness

Glycerine and lemon juice in equal parts will quickly give back a lost voice. This mixture is quite palatable.

Influenza

A hot water bottle, wrapped in flannel, is to be placed in the bed of a sufferer from unfluenza as a foot warmer. Keep the head cool and the feet warm.

Insomnia

A good remedy for sleeplessness is to drink hot water. If you awake in the night and become hopelessly wide awake, the cure is to sip a glass of hot, not warm water.

Lettuce greatly helps people suffering from sleeplessness.

For sleeplessness try a glass of warm milk – not hot, for it is then a stimulant – at bedtime.

Soak a towel in water and lay it on the stomach.

Onions eaten at night are a wonderful antidote for insomnia.

Insomnia is caused by the blood vessels in the brain being overcharged, and this may be prevented by a hot footbath the last thing at night.

If one suffers from insomnia, then an abundant use of lettuce is the cure. Lettuce is full of opium, a sleep giver, a nerve soother and rest inducer. It is not necessary to eat all the lettuce leaf, though the greenstuff is a blood purifier, the tender stem full of the milky juice, sliced up and eaten as a salad will be sufficient.

The onion too is a sleep bringer, a sudorific as well as a soporific. If a chill has been taken the eating of raw onions will drive it out, induce perspiration and bring sleep.

Jaundice

Lemon juice is beneficial in cases of jaundice from sluggishness of the biliary functions.

Leg Cramps.

It is a good plan when there is a tendency to cramp to lie in bed well covered, and, if necessary, apply hot water bottles to induce perspiration. Friction with the hand upon the surface of the skin where the pain lies is good to promote action.

Liver

Carrots possess valuable antiseptic properties, which may be used internally or externally. Internally carrots are of great service in derangements of the liver.

Loss of Appetite

Raw onions are excellent blood purifiers as they contain sulphur. Copious doses of onions will bring much sulphur into the body, alter all its noxious acids and vitalise the blood wonderfully. For sulphur is an alterative; it is a salt that will join with other salts, making sulphates of them, so driving all present acids into new and beneficial combinations. To those who have lost appetite, therefore, onions are recommended, they will renew the wish for food.

Mouth Wash

A mouth wash of salt and cold water used once a day will harden sensitive gums and prevent soreness and bleeding.

Muscular Pains

Arnica tincture is a remedy used to help with muscular pains, it helps reduce swelling.

Nausea

Bicarbonate of soda is an excellent remedy for nausea. A saltspoonful taken in warm water, when first the attack is felt to be approaching, will often ward it off. It is a mistake to take lemon and baking soda. That just makes an effervescent drink, and has little or no effect. Baking soda, taken every morning in water, will do much to prevent a recurrence of these attacks.

Neck

Stiff neck can be speedily cured by rubbing it with oil camphorated oil or mustard is good, and wrapping in hot flannel.

Pain Relief

Anodynes relieve pain, lessen the excitability of nerves. Onions, sage, hops, scullcaps and valerian.

Pancreas

Antibilious correct the secretion of bile. Apples, grapes, lemons, red gooseberries, tomatoes, carrots, silver beet, centuary, dandelion, gentian.

Pneumonia

If sharp pains in the regions of the lungs, hot onion poultices put on one after the other until the patient is relieved are more efficacious than mustard plasters. The onions should be sliced and fried in lard until soft then put into a little woollen bag. Place this over the seat of pain just as hot as the patient can bear it, and have another bag ready to change with as soon as the first grows luke-warm. Keep this treatment up until the patient is relieved. When the pain has ceased apply greased cloths and cover with a good thick layer of cotton batting. This should be worn several days as a protection against further cold, the greased cloth being changed daily.

Rheumatism

Celery is splendid for those suffering from rheumatism. Spinach is also good for rheumatism.

Anyone suffering from rheumatism should wear woollen clothing always next to the skin, and be very careful never to get the feet wet or sit in damp clothes. If very thirsty – which is sometimes the case with rheumatism – drink only milk and soda – no stimulants. Try rubbing the body night and morning with a rough towel.

Eat mangoes in large quantities to help cure rheumatism.

Just before retiring at night, eat an apple for a period of two weeks which should help rheumatism.

Sour oranges are highly recommended for rheumatism.

Shingles

A medicinal tincture of the common buttercup, if taken in small doses and applied, will promptly and effectively cure the troublesome ailment known as shingles, while it will further serve to banish a neuralgic or rheumatic stitch occurring in the side from any cause.

Watercress will cure scurvy.

Sore Throat

Gargling hot water, as hot as the throat will tolerate is an excellent remedy, especially when there is inflammation or irritation of the membrane at the back. In acute cases this is said to give immediate relief. In chronic, long-standing throat troubles, it will benefit, if preserved in.

A gargle of hot water and a small quantity of table salt is very good for sore throats.

Vinegar and water make a good gargle for a sore throat.

One of the oldest of country remedies for a sore throat is mulled elderberry wine, concocted from the fruit with raisins, sugar, and spices. Its efficacy has been attested by generations, and science has provided the explanation that elderberries furnish viburnic acid, a substance which induces sweating and is especially curative of inflammatory bronchial soreness.

A raw egg swallowed whole will often carry down a fishbone which is stuck in the throat.

Sores

As a poultice, the carrot, boiled and mashed into a pulp, is unrivalled for cleansing sores, sweetening and healing them.

Spasms

Antispasmodics relieve spasms, by exerting a stimulating action throughout the entire system, especially on the nervous system, which they sooth, without over stimulation. Celery, lettuce, thyme, cayenne, anise, fennel, aromatics, herbs such as carraway.

Sprains

Hot water is an excellent remedy for sprained joints. Immerse the joint in as hot water as can be borne, repeating often, the more often the better. Inflammation is always benefited by hot water.

Wormwood boiled in vinegar and applied as hot as can be taken on a sprain is an invaluable remedy.

Stings

Salt mixed with common washing soda is an excellent cure for stings.

Stomach

Antracids reduce acidity of the stomach. Apples, bananas, barley, slippery elm.

Stomach Cramps

For sudden pain or cramp in the stomach, hot water treatment is beneficial. If this is not effectual, pour a cupful of boiling water upon a teaspoonful of ginger. Let it stand a few minutes, and drink it. An ordinary pain or cramp will yield to this.

For a pain in the stomach, try some pepper in a glass of hot water.

Sunburn

For a sunburnt neck good remedy applied several times a day is lemon juice and lime water in equal parts.

Teeth

The toothbrush is not sufficiently cleansed by being rinsed in hot and cold water. Keep a phial bottle on your basin containing a solution of boric acid, and twice a week, after rinsing the toothbrush dip it into a little boric solution and hot water. Stand for a few minutes, then shake out and dry. A few drops of the boric acid solution on the toothbrush will keep the teeth and gums healthy.

Cloves are good to relieve toothache.

For toothache you boil sandalwood leaves in water and then put some of the juice in the cavity of the aching tooth.

Another possible help for toothache is to put a pinch of bicarbonate of soda in the mouth, take a mouthful of water and well rinse the teeth. If the pain is in one tooth, get a piece of cotton wool, wet it, smear it with the soda, and place in the cavity. If this is done in time a bad toothache may be averted.

Rubbing mustard behind the ear will often ease toothache.

Teething

When babies are teething they suffer very much from thirst, which is caused by feverishness. To allay the thirst it is a good plan to give a teaspoonful or two of pure cold water several times during the day. It is wonderful how this will soothe fretful babies when everything else has failed.

Thrush

For the treatment of thrush a solution of borax or bicarbonate of soda – one fourth teaspoonful to a pint of water.

Tonsils

After a severe attack of tonsillitis, the throat is often relaxed, and the tonsils still quite painful. An old fashioned remedy still in use in many parts of the West of England is a conserve of roses. This is a sort of jam made from the hips of the common wild rose. It is not unpleasant in taste and certainly possesses strongly astringent properties. Another village remedy is the juice of the mulberry squeezed into warm water and slightly sweetened. This is given to children who wake at night with feverish thirst. Mulberry juice has a curious property of quenching thirst.

A gargle made of a teaspoonful of powdered tannin dissolved in a tumbler of water and used every two hours relieves swollen tonsils.

Tuberculous

Watercress juice can help with tuberculous, it is chemically rich in anti-scorbutic salts, which tend to possibly destroy the germs of tuberculous.

Ulcers

Paw paw can help cure ulcers. Make an ointment consisting of lard and paw paw juice.

Varicose Veins

For varicose veins rub the leg upwards for five minutes every night and morning.

Warts

Salicylic acid is the infallible cure for warts or rub them with an apple.

THE END

References

1928 'SIMPLE REMEDIES', *Sunday Times (Perth, WA : 1902 - 1954)*, 1 January, p. 29. , viewed 21 Jan 2017, http://nla.gov.au/nla.news-article60305076

1925 'Homely Remedies', *The Daily Mail (Brisbane, Qld. : 1903 - 1926)*, 18 October, p. 20. , viewed 21 Jan 2017, http://nla.gov.au/nla.news-article220635933

1901 'HOME REMEDIES.', *Examiner (Launceston, Tas. : 1900 - 1954)*, 3 August, p. 3. (DAILY.), viewed 21 Jan 2017, http://nla.gov.au/nla.news-article91660906

1916 'REMEDIES.', *The Ballarat Star (Vic. : 1865 - 1924)*, 24 June, p. 9. , viewed 21 Jan 2017, http://nla.gov.au/nla.news-article154671917

1925 'Homely Remedies.', *The Daily Mail (Brisbane, Qld. : 1903 - 1926)*, 3 May, p. 20. , viewed 21 Jan 2017, http://nla.gov.au/nla.news-article218248851

1906 'DOMESTIC REMEDIES', *The Sunday Sun (Sydney, NSW : 1903 - 1910)*, 2 September, p. 11. , viewed 21 Jan 2017, http://nla.gov.au/nla.news-article231864846

1927 'SIMPLE REMEDIES', *Northern Star (Lismore, NSW : 1876 - 1954)*, 3 September, p. 15. , viewed 21 Jan 2017, http://nla.gov.au/nla.news-article93641028

1940 'BUSH REMEDIES', *Chronicle (Adelaide, SA : 1895 - 1954)*, 14 November, p. 34. , viewed 21 Jan 2017, http://nla.gov.au/nla.news-article92399558

1901 'HOME MEDICINE CHEST.', *Western Mail (Perth, WA : 1885 - 1954)*, 22 June, p. 65. , viewed 21 Jan 2017, http://nla.gov.au/nla.news-article33207023

1904 'Science.', *Narandera Argus and Riverina Advertiser (NSW : 1893 - 1953)*, 8 April, p. 6. , viewed 21 Jan 2017, http://nla.gov.au/nla.news-article130449878

1945 'Homely Remedies', *Townsville Daily Bulletin (Qld. : 1907 - 1954)*, 7 August, p. 6. , viewed 21 Jan 2017, http://nla.gov.au/nla.news-article62857317

1914 'DOMESTIC REMEDIES', *The Mail (Adelaide, SA : 1912 - 1954)*, 31 January, p. 3. , viewed 21 Jan 2017, http://nla.gov.au/nla.news-article59642341

1916 'Nature Cures.', *Spectator and Methodist Chronicle (Melbourne, Vic. : 1914 - 1918)*, 4 August, p. 1006. , viewed 21 Jan 2017, http://nla.gov.au/nla.news-article154269613

1902 'KITCHEN REMEDIES.', *The Evening Star (Boulder, WA : 1898 - 1921)*, 12 August, p. 4. , viewed 22 Jan 2017, http://nla.gov.au/nla.news-article202859761

1906 'DOMESTIC REMEDIES.', *The Sunday Sun (Sydney, NSW : 1903 - 1910)*, 29 July, p. 11. , viewed 22 Jan 2017, http://nla.gov.au/nla.news-article231865389

1974 'The best cure for a hangover', *The Beverley Times (WA : 1905 - 1977)*, 14 March, p. 4. , viewed 22 Jan 2017, http://nla.gov.au/nla.news-article202741344

1939 'Simple Cures.', *The Catholic Press (Sydney, NSW : 1895 - 1942)*, 22 June, p. 4. , viewed 22 Jan 2017, http://nla.gov.au/nla.news-article106367871

1913 'FRUIT AS MEDICINE.', *Evening News (Sydney, NSW : 1869 - 1931)*, 30 January, p. 5. , viewed 22 Jan 2017, http://nla.gov.au/nla.news-article113781623

1906 'DOMESTIC REMEDIES', *The Sunday Sun (Sydney, NSW : 1903 - 1910)*, 9 December, p. 7. , viewed 22 Jan 2017, http://nla.gov.au/nla.news-article231877703

1971 'Cure for hangover', *The Beverley Times (WA : 1905 - 1977)*, 21 January, p. 7. , viewed 22 Jan 2017, http://nla.gov.au/nla.news-article202738432

1949 'WATER A CURE FOR HANGOVER', *Tweed Daily (Murwillumbah, NSW : 1914 - 1949)*, 8 March, p. 3. , viewed 22 Jan 2017, http://nla.gov.au/nla.news-article194563800

1950 'MANY CURES GIVEN FOR THAT HANGOVER', *Barrier Miner (Broken Hill, NSW : 1888 - 1954)*, 24 July, p. 3. , viewed 22 Jan 2017, http://nla.gov.au/nla.news-article49593526

1957 'HERE'S YOUR CURE', *The Argus (Melbourne, Vic. : 1848 - 1957)*, 1 January, p. 3. , viewed 22 Jan 2017, http://nla.gov.au/nla.news-article71773998

1902 'KITCHEN MEDICINE.', *Examiner (Launceston, Tas. : 1900 - 1954)*, 24 May, p. 3. (DAILY.), viewed 22 Jan 2017, http://nla.gov.au/nla.news-article35487568